I0422042

Cure Back Pain Naturally

By Kishora Patel

Special Edition, License Notes

This book is licensed for your personal use only. This book may not be re-sold or given away to other people. If you would like to share this book with another person, please purchase an additional copy for each recipient. If you're reading this book and did not purchase it, or it was not purchased for your use only, then please purchase your own copy.

Cure Back Pain Naturally

Copyright © Kishora Patel 2015

First published 2015

Special Edition

All rights reserved. Without limiting the rights under copyright reserved above, no part of this publication may be reproduced, stored in or introduced into a database and retrieval system or transmitted in any form or any means (electronic, mechanical, photocopying, recording or otherwise) without the prior written permission of both the owner of copyright and the above publishers.

Cure Back Pain Naturally

Patel, Kishora

Table of Contents

Introduction

As we move through the early years of the new century, the pace of every day life is becoming ever more frantic. With every passing day, there appears to be more to get done than there ever was before. At the same time, there is little doubt that the strain of modern day life has the tendency to keep on increasing instead of declining and enabling us to relax in the way that we would probably all prefer to.

Because life is turning out to be increasingly more frantic and challenging, there is certainly little doubt that the tensions and stresses on your body are also increasing on an everyday basis. It is little surprise that a great number of people are plagued with persistent niggles, aches and pains. Indeed, some unfortunate folks are compelled to suffer their discomfort in silence, seeking to live a life which is as normal as is possible. Of course, because most people do not find themselves in this particular situation, they almost certainly give very little thought or maybe no thought at all to the pummeling that their body takes everyday. That is likely to continue until some kind of serious pain strikes, and from that point on, pain becomes a very real and important concern in their life.

Some varieties of pain are less serious than others, and many types of discomfort will come and go. However, not every pain issue can be so simply dismissed and amongst those that are most commonly felt and painfully endured is back pain.

It is estimated that between 50 million and 80 million US citizens have problems with persistent pain (defined as a pain that has lasted for longer than six months), and that this costs over $100 billion in social costs annually. Back pain is one of the most common causes of men and women going to their doctor or medical practitioner.

Without a doubt, it has been estimated that upwards of four out of every five people in the world are going to need to consult a medical professional at some stage in their lives with a back pain problem. For those who have never suffered back pain, it is possible that they may sympathize with those that are frequent sufferers, but it is unlikely that they can really appreciate the amount of pain and suffering that back pain brings. Only a fellow back pain sufferer can really sympathize and empathize with other sufferers who have been stricken with an identical problem to theirs.

It is also relevant to note that the prevalence of persistent back pain issues is on the increase, and that there are undoubtedly a lot more sufferers nowadays than there have ever been at any previous time in history. However, one undeniable fact is that anyone who has ever suffered from back pain, or (even worse) knows just how much misery and suffering the affliction can bring. These individuals would do just about anything to try to find a non-invasive remedy or treatment for their condition.

As with any medical condition, it is better and therefore preferable to deal with back pain in a natural manner whenever possible, and that is the fundamental topic of this book. What exactly is back pain, and what causes it? What is the best way to deal with it?

What Is Back Pain?

Stating the obvious, back pain is a pain or discomfort that you feel in your back, with the most common form being pain or discomfort in the lower back area. Most importantly, it is an indication that there is something wrong with your back, usually something that is related to musculoskeletal problems.

The problem for most people that suffer back pain is that they never give it a moment's thought most of the time, because during those periods of their life they are not in pain. However, as soon as the pain hits, it is a pain that they will feel almost irrespective of what they are doing. If they are walking or standing, they will be in pain, but even if they are sitting down in a favorite chair or lying down, the chances are that they will still feel the pain.

For anyone who is lucky enough to suffer back pain only intermittently, they will forget how much difficulty they were previously suffering after the pain has gone away again.

The complaint of lower back pain is one of the most common medical complaints known, and yet, because there are many possible causes, it can also be one of the most frustrating and difficult problems for both patients and their medical attendants to deal with. The good news is that for most people, back problems do tend to be intermittent - meaning that they are likely to go away of their own volition given time. The amount of time will depend upon the condition itself, the severity of the pain and so on, but for most people, having a 'bad back' is a temporary problem.

It is generally believed that once you have suffered a back problem, you become more prone to suffering similar problems again in the future. It is for this reason that even an intermittent, temporary back problem can become a major difficulty for anyone who works in a profession where lifting is essential for them to fulfill the tasks of their job. As an example, it can be a major career threat for anyone in the nursing profession to suffer a damaged back, because it is absolutely necessary for them to be able to help patients up from a prone position, which necessitates lifting.

What Causes Back Pain?

A simple answer to this question is it is probably your life that is causing your back pain problem. Using the previous nursing profession example, it is common for back problems to first blight nursing staff because they have made the mistake of lifting a heavier than average patient in the wrong way.

This gives one pointer to a primary cause of back pain for many people. They suffer such pain as a direct side effect of the life they lead, or, more specifically, they often suffer as a 'side effect' of the job that they do.

It is a fact that your lower back bears most of the weight of your upper body, and consequently, most back pain occurs as a result of using incorrect lifting techniques leading to strained back muscles and sprained ligaments. Alternatively, it is very common for these sorts of problems to be caused by an individual making a sudden, jarring movement that jolts their back and damages a muscle.

You may suffer a back spasm, or build up stress in a particular part of your back over a period of time that only needs the proverbial straw to break (or at least damage) your back.

Hence, if you have a back pain that you did not have yesterday, the first thing to suspect is that you did something yesterday to cause this pain. It does not need to be something that is particularly strenuous or difficult, and it is not always obvious what the root cause of your pain might be.

For example, it is a fact of modern life that more and more of us spend hours every day sitting at a desk in front of a computer. Unfortunately, your spine is not well designed for hours of physical inactivity sitting hunched over a computer keyboard, and it is therefore feasible that this single activity could be just as damaging to your back as would be lifting an over-heavy object.

It is for this reason that if you are deskbound and working in front of a computer, you should make an effort to stand at least once every hour, and if you can have a short wander round, that makes things even better. Even when you are sitting down, try to change your position and shift your body weight whenever possible, because it is the inactivity of not doing so that can adversely affect your back and cause pain.

A similar proviso would apply to any one who spends several hours a day behind the wheel of their car or truck. Take regular breaks, have a stroll about, and remember to shift your weight as regularly as possible while you are behind the wheel.

If you are unfortunate enough to wake up in the morning with a back pain, it is unlikely that you are going to be able to make the necessary changes to your daily routine immediately. However, once the pain has abated, that is the time to make changes to your routine. Focus in particular on those aspects of your daily activities that might have caused the initial back problem.

While there are obviously specific medical conditions that cause back pain (we will consider these in the next section), more often than not intermittent back pain is caused by a specific aspect of your daily routine or lifestyle.

In this scenario, it should not be difficult to isolate exactly what has caused the problem for most people, and therefore it should also be easy to make the changes necessary to prevent the problem coming back again.

For most people, their bad back condition is only likely to last a few days or a couple of weeks at the outside. In this case, prevention of a re-occurrence is largely down to being able to pinpoint what caused your bad back in the first place, and making the necessary changes to ensure that the same situation does not arise again in the future.

Of course, there may be more to it than simply making a small change in your lifestyle.

For example, if you are seriously overweight, this fact significantly increases the chances of you suffering back pain. As your spine and lower back supports your body weight, there is simply too much weight for it to do so properly.

In this case, the only answer that is going to be effective in the longer term is to reduce your weight significantly. Unfortunately, this is not likely to be a speedy process, on the basis that if you are carrying enough excess weight to cause a back problem, it is likely to take some time to shift that excess weight.

Similarly, if the cause of your current back pain problem was an accident (e. g. whiplash injuries from a motor vehicle accident), then you may have suffered long-term damage that is going to require a significant degree of medical treatment in order to effect a cure.

Obviously, no-one has a major accident deliberately, and therefore lifestyle changes are not going to address the root cause of the problem.

Medical Causes Of Back Pain

Lumbar muscle strains:

Strains of the muscles in the lower back are by far and away the most common cause of back pain, and most of the back pain problems that we have already considered in this report would probably fall into this category.

A muscle strain is a rip or a tear in the muscle fibers that is caused by sudden force.

Consequently, whilst there may be a single, sudden cause of such a strain, it is equally possible that there will be no single event upon which you can blame your condition. You could have strained your lumbar muscles lifting something that was too heavy or lifting it in the incorrect manner, but you could equally have caused the condition by sitting in a chair or even lying in your bed in an awkward manner.

The good news is, lumbar muscle strains will almost certainly go away quickly, and you will not necessarily be any more prone to a repeat 'attacks' after the strain has cleared up than is anyone else.

Alternatively, it is relatively common to suffer a back sprain, which is caused by an overstretching of one or more of the ligaments in your back. Whilst strains and sprains are therefore different conditions, they are generally treated in the same way when it comes to alleviating the pain caused by either condition.

Disc problems:

The human spine runs down the centre of the back from the skull to the pelvis, and is comprised of 33 individual vertebrae. These vertebrae are categorized into four different groups as indicated in the screenshot.

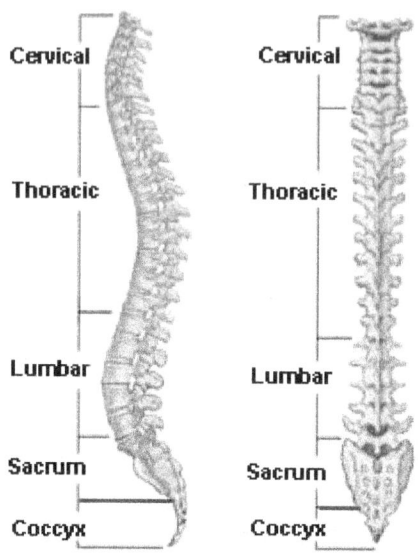

In between each of these individual vertebrae you will find a small disc which is made up of a tough outer coating (the annulus), and a gel-like central interior (the nucleus pulposus). These discs are designed to act as 'shock absorbers' between each of the vertebrae which in turn enables your spine to flex, bend and move in a controlled manner while not causing you any discomfort or pain (under normal circumstances).

Quite clearly however, if any of the 'shock absorbing' discs have a problem, then the vertebrae of your spine are likely to knock together or jar one another, and this will often cause a great deal of pain.

One disc related condition that you may suffer from is a slipped disc. This happens when the soft gel like interior of the disc pushes itself out through the tough outer coating - with two possible results, either of which may (but may not) cause you pain. Firstly, you no longer have a 'shock absorber' between your vertebrae, and secondly, the escaped gel-like substance may put additional pressure on your spinal-cord or the nerve cells in that area, in which case, you will undoubtedly feel a great deal of pain.

However, it is important to note that, whether you feel pain or not, if the nucleus pulposus has escaped from a disc in your spine, then you have a slipped disc, irrespective of whether there is any pain or not.

Sometimes, you will suffer what is known as a ruptured (or herniated) disk which is pretty much the same as happens with a slipped disc. However, the phrase is most commonly used in connection with the lumbar and cervical vertebrae, primarily the former.

These are the five vertebrae that do most of the supporting work of the spine, and consequently the pressure on these particular vertebrae is considerable.

Again, you have a ruptured lumber disc when the soft gel-like substance from inside the disc escapes through the tough outer coating of the disc.

As we get older, the discs in our spine become less pliable, so it therefore becomes increasingly likely that you will suffer a slipped or ruptured disc.

Sciatica:

Sciatica is another relatively common form of back pain. This is a term that is used to describe a pain that not only affects the lower back, but also stretches down into the buttocks and legs. It results from irritation or overstimulation of a large nerve in the spinal column known as the sciatic nerve. Because sciatica is a pain that is associated with irritation of a particular nerve, it is a condition that can accompany other less serious back problems like muscle strains and ligament sprains.

Spinal stenosis:

This is another condition that is associated with getting older. The spinal column itself can become more restrictive as a result of a condition like arthritis, and as a result it can put pressure on the spinal cord or surrounding nerves. In this case, pain is the almost inevitable result.

Osteoporosis:

This is another condition that is generally associated with the ageing process, one in which the bones throughout the body get continually weaker due to reduced levels of calcium. Consequently, because the bones are gradually weakening, it is not uncommon to find osteoporosis has caused compression fractures of the vertebrae, particularly in older women.

Lumbar spine arthritis: Although it is likely that you are most familiar with arthritis as a medical condition that mainly affects external parts of the body such as the fingers, hands and toes, it is a fact that arthritis can attack any bone and joint in the body. Consequently, arthritis can attack the joints in the spine, making almost any kind of movement a very painful process.

Spondylolisthesis: When adjacent vertebrae in the spine become unstable because of a general degenerative condition in that area of the body, individual vertebrae can begin to shift their positions relative to one another. In this scenario, it is always possible that individual vertebrae will start grinding or rubbing against one another, and this will cause a great deal of back pain.

Medical Treatments For Back Pain.

Although this book is focused on natural treatments for back problems, it should be obvious from the range of medical conditions that can cause back pain that natural treatments are not capable of curing every problem that might cause such pain.

For example, anti-inflammatory drugs (more commonly known as non- specific anti-inflammatory drugs) can sometimes be useful for reducing the pain in your back, and also bringing down any associated inflammation. However, like all pharmaceutical drugs, even NSAIDs can have side-effects such as an increased risk of gastro-intestinal bleeding. Thus, they are not ideal for everyone who suffers from a back pain problem, and they should be taken for as short a period of time as possible.

In addition, there are narcotic pain killers that will reduce the pain symptoms, but they can also be used only for a limited period of time with any degree of safety. Drug based muscle relaxants might also be prescribed by your medical attendant if the primary cause of your back pain problems is muscle spasms. In this case, however, muscle relaxants (such as Valium) are likely to make you drowsy, so once again, great care has to be applied if you intend to take such drugs.

If you are suffering from inflammation around the spinal nerves, your medical practitioner may recommend an epidural steroid injection that will reduce both the pain and the inflammation around the nerves at the same time. Steroids are another pharmaceutical drug that you should only take for a limited period of time, and most people who have had an epidural will tell you that it is no walk in the park!

The final solution is spinal surgery, but this actually only happens in a small number of cases. Spinal surgery only becomes necessary after trying all other treatments without success, hence it is most commonly used as a treatment of last resort.

Spinal surgery is only really effective for a limited number of conditions listed in the previous section such as spondylolisthesis, spinal stenosis or to remove a ruptured disc should that become necessary (which is unusual).

Most physicians will only consider surgery when they believe that the risk of not undertaking surgery is greater than the risk of doing so. For example, if after a considerable period of non-invasive treatment, a slipped or ruptured disc is not getting any better, it can quite easily start to get worse. In this situation, it is possible that spinal surgery will be considered. Balanced against this, there is always a risk involved in such surgical procedures, specifically the risk of paralysis, because this is surgery undertaken in very close proximity to the individual patient's spinal cord. Surgery is generally only considered when all else has failed and the situation is clearly deteriorating.

Beyond this short list of recognized medical treatments for various causes of back pain and associated problems, there are many natural treatments that you can apply to reduce the severity of your back pain, and to treat your condition at the same time.

Before starting to look at these natural treatments in greater detail, however, let me first set out what I would consider to be a sensible approach to consulting a qualified member of the medical profession about your back pain problem.

When To Consider Seeking Medical Attention.

As suggested, the majority of back problems that most people suffer from are likely to be caused by muscle strains of one form or another. In this situation, it is unlikely that there will be any need for serious medical attention or treatment.

While not belittling the fact that back muscle strains can be very painful indeed, there is very little that your medical practitioner can do to help you in this situation other than prescribing painkillers and relieving creams or ointments. Unless you know that these are 100% natural, you may not want to take or use them in any event.

If you have a new case of back pain that you cannot explain, you may want to contact your medical practitioner for an evaluation.

However, there are certain situations where you should definitely seek medical attention for your back pain, because it may be that it is a symptom or an indication of something that might be more serious. In particular, make sure that you contact your doctor if:

• The pain lasts more than a week or so, and does not seem to be decreasing in severity;

• You have a back pain that is accompanied with an inability to properly control your bladder or bowels;

• You have chills, fevers. sweating, trembling or find that you feel alternately hot and cold. In this case, you have a fever as well as back pain, which clearly needs checking at the soonest opportunity;

• You notice any other unusual additional symptoms that would not normally be associated with a muscle strain or ligament sprain.

The Difficulty With Back Problems.

If you were to be in a position to ask any suitably qualified member of the medical profession, you would probably be reliably informed that understanding and diagnosing back problems is one of the most frustrating and difficult tasks any member of the medical profession will ever face.

The problem that they face is that unless there is a clear clinical, medical condition (such as osteoporosis) which can give them a clue as to the root cause of your back problems, it can be very difficult for any medical practitioner to come up with a categorical explanation of your back problems.

If you are a person who very rarely has a back problem, or you are in a position to pinpoint a particular activity that has probably strained your back, the medical professional who you consult is not likely to have much of a problem diagnosing and/or treating your problem.

On the other hand, if you have a long-term or persistent back pain problem, then you should adopt a different approach if you choose to consult a medical professional (and there is absolutely no harm at all in seeking professional opinion).

In this case, expecting an informed medical opinion the very first time you consult with a new medical adviser is simply not realistic.

Given that diagnosing back problems is notoriously difficult, if you expect an answer immediately, you are likely to make a mistake that many back pain sufferers make. This is the error of 'jumping' from one medical professional to another on an almost never-ending basis in the desperate hope that someone is going to come up with a miracle diagnosis for your problem.

This is not the way it works in the real world. What you need to do is to find a medical practitioner with whom you are comfortable – an orthopedist, osteopath or general medical practitioner – and work with them for a period of at least several weeks, and ideally several months.

By doing things in this way, you give them a realistic chance of discovering what your real problem is. This enables them to treat your condition in the most appropriate manner, although you should not expect an instant, miracle cure, because it may well be that no such thing exists even after they have discovered the root cause of your problem.

Only if you have given them sufficient time and you still find that they can come up with no satisfactory answer should you consider moving on to seek someone else's opinion.

A Rest Is As Good As A Cure.

Perhaps surprisingly, one of the most obvious natural treatments for back pain is also one of the most effective. Even if you are suffering from something as apparently serious as a slipped disc, it is quite likely that your medical practitioner will recommend flat bed rest as the first cause of treatment.

It is also likely that he or she will also prescribe inflammatory drugs and painkillers as well, but, as previously suggested, you probably don't want to take these if you are looking for a natural cure for your back pain problems. Moreover, the fact the bed rest is considered to be a practical treatment for such an apparently serious condition should give you some indication of how highly rated rest is as a back pain treatment, and there could be nothing more natural than rest.

Even if you have nothing more than a muscle strain, bed rest is a great way of reducing the severity of the pain, but you should not stay in bed for more than two or three days, because doing so can actually make the pain worse rather than better.

Knowing this, the next thing that you must know is that your choice of bed is an absolutely critical factor in how much back pain relief you will get from flat bed rest. However, this does not necessarily mean that you should invest in a bed that is described as having any particular medical properties, or as an orthopedic bed or mattress.

In fact, according to research in the UK, the majority of orthopedic mattresses are too hard, and as a result, only 6% of experts would recommend an orthopedic mattress to back pain sufferers.

What you are looking for is a bed mattress that is firm and supportive, as opposed to being hard. Furthermore, if you are a regular back pain sufferer, you should also consider changing your bed more frequently, because older beds and mattresses are less likely to give you the support and comfort that you need to alleviate or perhaps even get rid of your back condition.

There would also be an argument here for spending as much money as you can afford on your next bed if you are a constant back pain sufferer, because it does seem from all available research that sleeping in or on a high-quality bed can make a significant difference to your back pain problems.

Obviously, everyone who suffers a back pain condition has a slightly different problem and therefore there is not one ideal sleeping solution that covers every back pain sufferer. For this reason, you must be willing to do a little research when you buy your next bed. That bed could be the difference between your continuing to suffer back problems for as long as you sleep in it, or solving your problems in a matter of weeks.

No matter where you live, your local bed store will offer dozens of choices, but do not be persuaded by a sales person to take the bed that they believe is best for your back problems ('but everyone who has a back problem buys the Super-ABC bed!').

Find beds that seem to have the appropriate degree of firmness and support, and test every one for at least 10 minutes in your normal sleeping position. Do this and your back will very soon tell you whether you are looking at the right bed or not!

Is the bed the right height for you to get in and out without any back pain or discomfort? If it is so low or so high that entry and exit are likely to exacerbate your back problems, you should move on to the next option immediately.

Buy as big a bed as you can afford, particularly if there are two people going to share it. This ensures that you or both of you have plenty of room to move, which should help with a good night's sleep.

Finally, do take time to consider the pillows that you use, and how many of them you generally sleep with. If your pillows are too high, they could significantly alter the shape and angle of your body during sleep, and if your shape is not good, this could offset the benefits that you hope to gain by getting a new bed in the first place.

Also, think about your individual sleeping position, and try to find one that appears to put the least strain on your back.

Lose Weight And Get Fitter.

As with any medical condition, rather than waiting for a back pain problem to develop, it makes far more sense to take steps before you ever suffer the first invidious twinges of back pain to take steps to ensure that you never do so.

One way that you could do this has already been mentioned earlier in this report. If you are overweight or obese, you are at a significantly higher risk of suffering back problems and therefore you should begin to shed the extra weight as soon as possible.

Of course, this will not only benefit your back, as your general health is also likely to increase significantly as you shed the extra bulk that is undoubtedly putting a strain on your general health and well-being. For example, your heart will undoubtedly be working harder than it really needs to do if you are significantly overweight or obese, and you are at a far higher risk of suffering diabetes than you would otherwise be.

Add these to the fact that losing weight is going to take a great strain off your spine, and doing so becomes something of an no-brainer!

However, even if you are not at all overweight or obese, you may not be as fit and a strong as you could otherwise be. This is significant, because, if for example, you start working out at the gym once or twice a week, you will improve your muscle tone, strength and flexibility over time. This improved strength and flexibility will naturally make it considerably less likely that you will suffer back strains, for example.

This is not to suggest that you need to become a body builder or weightlifter or that you need to go to the gym every day. However, it is a fact that the more flexible, strong and fit you are, the less likely it becomes that you will suffer the strains or pulls that are the most common cause of back pain complaints.

Moreover, you are going to significantly reduce the chances of suffering other muscle injuries by becoming fitter and stronger, and your general ability to deal with minor medical problems will also be enhanced.

Prevention is always better than having to find a cure, and in the case of the most common cause of back pain complaints, prevention is to a very large extent in your own hands.

There are other ways in which a 'workout' based exercise program can help reduce the chances of suffering back problems in the future.

For example, it is generally believed that weight-bearing exercise helps to reduce the bone loss that is a primary symptom of osteoporosis, as well as keeping muscles toned which can again help to offset the worst effects of osteoporosis.

In this respect, basic exercises like walking, playing tennis or aerobics can be a big help, particularly for women who are the primary sufferers of osteoporosis.

Insufficient calcium in your diet also increases the chances of suffering the bone wasting disease, which would in turn increase the chances of suffering back problems in later life.

Vitamin D deficiency also increases the probability of suffering fractures, and this is another condition which gets worse as you get older. Vitamin D is generally generated by the body through the action of sunlight on the skin, but it is possible to supplement your diet in order to make sure that you take enough on board.

Prolonged use of tobacco and/or alcohol can also increase your chances of contracting osteoporosis later in life. Once again, it comes down to the notion of living a healthy life in order to prevent unpleasant or even potentially crippling medical conditions (remember that osteoporosis makes your bones more susceptible to fracture, and a snapped spine often equals paralysis) later in life.

Not All Back Problems Are Minor

Many people who have the biggest back problems, those that suffer the greatest degree of pain, are people whose condition has nothing to do with a minor muscle strain, nor have they suffered any of the medical ailments highlighted earlier in this book.

These are people who have suffered spinal injury, and for many of these people, it can be a very long and hard road back to full fitness and normality, if they are ever fortunate enough to regain that condition.

For such people, the initial treatment usually involves a degree of necessary medical treatment to 'patch them up' in the early stages. However, once the surgeons have 'done their magic', it is interesting to note that the job of bringing these people back to as close to normality as they can ever hope to be is almost always entrusted to people who employ natural means and strategies to do their job.

As some of these strategies could have a part to play in reducing pain for anyone who has a particularly serious back problem (however it is caused), it may help to look at some of the more practical back pain solutions.

Physical therapists: These are trained individuals whose job it is to work with anyone who has suffered injuries or surgery to return them to full activity, strength and mobility as quickly as possible. They will generally teach specialized exercises and techniques using equipment specially designed for the task, and they are trained to recognize deficiencies or weaknesses in the biomechanics of any individual patient's anatomy.

For example, a physical therapist will focus on stretching tight muscles and joints because without the ability to stretch, you naturally lose mobility. Furthermore, the stronger and more mobile you, the more you have the ability to fight against any joint or muscle pain, and that applies just as much to the muscles and joints in your back as it does to any other part of your body.

If the injury you have suffered necessitates an exercise program designed to strengthen the muscles of your back, then you would find many appropriate exercises in the pages below.

Aquatherapy & Ultrasound

Aquatherapy is equally exercise based as it would be if you were working with a physical therapist, with the main difference that your exercises are all carried out in water. The relevance of this is that when you are submerged in water, you become weightless, and it is therefore far easier to exercise without putting strain on your body or applying pressure to your muscles. Consequently, aquatherapy is a superb environment in which to work painful back muscles in order to loosen them and strengthen them in a non-impact environment.

For example, if you were recovering from a back injury and needed gentle traction (stretching), then you might find yourself hanging by the arms, being supported by a float with small weights attached to your legs.

Ultrasound: This is a form of high energy soundwave-based treatment that has many medical uses, including having the ability to help repair damaged muscles and bones while relieving the pain at the same time. Obviously, whilst it is unlikely that your medical attendant or physician would recommend ultrasound for a simple muscle strain, it is certainly something that could happen if you suffered serious accidental muscle injury.

Alternative Ways Of Getting Rid Of Back Pain.

As previously suggested, one very simple, effective but completely natural way of getting rid of your back pain is to stay in bed for a couple of days.

Alternatively, if you are already someone who suffers chronic back problem or perhaps someone who falls into a high risk category for back pain in the future, you should consider making whatever lifestyle changes are necessary so that you become stronger, fitter and healthier. In this way, you will reduce or completely remove the possibility of ever suffering back pain problems again.

This is all very well and good, but if you already have back pain, there is no doubt that you want to know how to get rid of it as quickly and effectively as possible. Furthermore, by the fact that you are reading this book, it is clear that you are looking for a natural back pain solution, which is what you are going to read about in the next few chapters.

The method of back pain relief that you seek will be very much dependent upon the cause of that back pain. If your back pain is caused by a serious medical condition (e. g. a fracture suffered as a result of osteoporosis or a slipped disc), then treating your back pain at home is not going to be an appropriate course of action.

However, given the fact that the majority of back pain problems will be caused by muscle strains or ligament pulls, we are going to focus on treatment that can be used to address pain caused by non-critical conditions.

In essence, if you have back pain caused by muscle strains or a pull, this is a situation that you can treat at home in a natural manner.

If it is anything worse, however, your back pain is likely to be something that requires medical treatment.

Heat And Ice Treatment.

Both heat and ice treatments can be used to deal with back pain from muscles, with the most suitable choice depending upon the reason for the pain.

If you have suffered some kind of back muscle injury, the first thing to ascertain is whether there is any swelling or inflammation. If there is no swelling, you are probably best advised to use heat to reduce the pain, because applying heat to a muscle increases its flexibility and elasticity.

Especially if activity is in the offing (even if it is only having to go to work), applying heat is probably more appropriate than applying an ice pack to your damaged muscles. In this way, you will encourage movement in your muscles, which is going to enable you to use them as and when it becomes necessary without suffering an undue degree of pain.

Because heat increases blood flow and skin temperature, you can apply an appropriate source of heat to your muscles for 15 to 20 minutes at a time. As moist heat is best, you could try using a hot towel or you could use a special athletic heat device or application on the injured area. There are also quite a few websites where you can buy natural heat applications like the National Allergy site.

Alternatively, there might be times when applying ice to your injury could be more appropriate. Although it is generally believed that applying an 'ice pack' of some description to any muscle injury is the best idea, heat works best for chronic pain.

If you are in the situation where your back pain is caused by an obvious injury where there may be swelling or inflammation, then application of an ice pack is likely to work better than applying a heat source. The application of ice acts as a vaso-constrictor, meaning that it will cause your blood vessels to narrow and that will limit internal bleeding and swelling.

Apply ice to the affected area (wrapped in a cloth or towel to prevent discomfort or 'ice burn') for 10 to 15 minutes at a time. After application, allow your skin temperature to return to normal before repeating the process as many times as necessary.

This is a process that you can repeat as many times as necessary for three or four days, but if after that, the problem still persists, you should seek appropriate medical advice.

If your back pain is caused by excess or unaccustomed physical activity or exercise, then the application of an ice pack may be the most appropriate solution. This is confirmed by the fact that cold therapy is often used by athletes who are trying to treat muscle pain caused by over-activity and the corresponding muscle stress.

If you have a back pain problem, the application of either heat or ice may well help to alleviate the severity of the pain.

After assessing the problem, decide which of the two alternatives seems most appropriate, whilst bearing in mind the fact that what is most suitable for one person will not necessarily be most appropriate for another.

You might need to test both alternatives, but if you do so, use cold therapy first because the application of heat could exacerbate any swelling or inflammation, whereas the application of ice tends to be more benign.

Eating For Back Pain Relief.

Perhaps surprisingly, athletes recognize that there are certain foods that you can take on board that can help to reduce or alleviate muscle pains. Of course, the pain relief benefits of eating certain foodstuffs could be as much psychological as they are physical, but it is not important how eating certain foods helps. If they help to relieve your back pain, then it really does not matter how that happens.

For instance, it may be that you suffer muscle pains in your back because of deficiencies in your diet, especially if your back pain is a result of exercise or activity to which you are not accustomed.

As an example, when you sweat, you tend to lose minerals and trace elements from your body, and if these minerals are not replaced you may suffer muscle pains and cramps.

A lack of both sodium and potassium can cause cramps and pain, but both can be replaced relatively quickly. Sodium can be ingested in bouillon (beef or chicken would be best, but a vegetable bouillon would also work), while bananas are a tremendous source of potassium.

Milk and milk-based dairy products are high in calcium, and calcium is essential for healthy bones and muscles. You should therefore drink a minimum of three glasses of milk a day if you are not taking on board sufficient calcium from other sources. This is particularly true of women who suffer back pain as a result of muscle strains or damage.

Depending upon the cause of your back pain, even plain water can be beneficial. This is especially true if your pain as a result of fluid depletion following exercise, but even if this is not the case, drinking water can help to alleviate back pain.

The bottom line is, you are supposed to drink at least eight glasses of water every day to maintain good health, so if you are not already doing so, now is the time to start, back pain or no back pain!

Back Pain, Traditional Chinese Medicine And Acupuncture.

In traditional Chinese medicine, there is no such thing as simple back pain. More correctly, there is not just one type of back pain but several, so that every individual back pain is classified and differentiated.

This is important to understand, because while acupuncture is widely recognized as being an effective treatment for back pain, the specific acupuncture points that would be used by a specialist would depend upon the type of pain from which you are suffering.

Amongst the different types of back pain recognized by traditional Chinese medicine, you will find:

• Deficiency type pain: This is a pain that is usually found in middle-aged or elderly people, one which is commonly characterized by a dull, aching pain that can be alleviated with rest.

• Blood stagnation or Qi ('energy flow') pain: In traditional Chinese medicine, it is believed that muscles are able to move blood, energy (Qi) and other bodily fluids by stretching and contracting. Consequently, if muscles are not stretched sufficiently strongly or often enough (which is true for most people in modern society), your Qi will become congested and it is likely that you will suffer significant or perhaps serious levels of pain.

• Cold and damp obstruction pain: This is a pain form that is most widely felt first thing in the morning, one that is made worse by the cold and damp weather. In Western medical terms, this would be the kind of pain most commonly associated with arthritis or sciatica. As would be expected with these particular medical conditions, this is a pain that is often accompanied by numbness, a feeling of weight or heaviness, and swelling in the joints or muscles of the back. Because this particular type of pain is exacerbated by the cold and damp, it is one that can be most effectively dealt with by the application of heat.

In traditional Chinese medicine, the basic concept is that when you feel any bodily pain or discomfort, it is telling you that your body balance and harmony is somehow upset. Consequently, in order to reduce or remove pain, it is necessary to restore balance and harmony and acupuncture is one of the primary modalities used to achieve this restoration. Acupuncture assumes that in modern society, most of us are not using (i.e. stretching and contracting) all of our muscles properly and that as a direct result of this disuse, many of our muscles have contracted and tightened.

This contraction and tightening means that Qi and blood are unable to flow through these muscles in the correct fashion, meaning that when we do try to use them, our muscles are simply not up to the task. Consequently, when an unusual strain is placed on the muscle in question (most commonly, the muscles of the lower back), that muscle will go into spasm even if this additional strain is relatively minor such as bending forward to pick something up from the floor or cleaning your teeth.

An acupuncturist will treat your back pain on the basis of moving blood and Qi around your body with the use of needles. A trained acupuncturist knows that there are many different blood and Qi 'channels' in your body, so their first task will be to palpitate various parts of your back to establish where the major centre points of pain are.

Points of pain are places where Qi has become congested, and the more pain there is, the more congestion there is assumed to be. As a result, the acupuncturist will insert needles in such a way that these channels are opened out so that the congestion and therefore the pain is removed.

Your acupuncture practitioner will apply needles in both a local (i. e. at the point of pain) and distal (i. e. in other parts of the body) manner in order to open up your Qi channels. Although it may appear to be somewhat counterintuitive, treating back pain using distal acupuncture points is very important, particularly in the treatment of acute back pain. Thus, needles placed in other parts of the body a considerable distance from the back can be extremely effective, although there are also many places in the back itself where acupuncture needles are likely to be extremely effective as well.

Alternatively, it is possible to enjoy acupuncture treatment where the practitioner uses an electric current rather than needles to stimulate the body and open the appropriate Qi channels. Given that many people have a fear or loathing of needles, this is often a more attractive alternative, although it may be more difficult to find a practitioner who will use electricity rather than needles.

The most important question is, does acupuncture work as a treatment for back pain? The results of a study conducted by two leading Swedish doctors in 2002 tend to indicate that the answer to the question appears to be an unqualified 'yes'.

According to the results published in 'The Clinical Journal of Pain' and reported on the Acupuncture Today website, the two doctors tested acupuncture as a back pain treatment on a group of people who had been suffering from chronic lower back pain for at least six months.

Every one of these people had tried various other back pain relief treatments or cures but to no avail.

The test group was split into three smaller groups. The members of one of these subgroups received acupuncture treatment once a week for eight weeks, the members of the second group received electro- acupuncture, and the members of the third subgroup were given a placebo.

The final results of the test indicated that all of the patients who had received acupuncture reported 'significant' improvement in their condition one month, three months and six months after completion of the treatment. They also reported that they were able to sleep more soundly than previously, and that they were also able to achieve higher activity levels than previously as well.

In short, there seems to be little doubt that acupuncture as a treatment for back pain can be extremely effective although the test did report that there were certain types of back pain and patients that responded to treatment better than others.

Perhaps most interestingly, the study also indicated that both forms of acupuncture (using needles or electro- acupuncture) were equally effective, indicating that even if you have a phobia about needles, acupuncture will still work for you if you are seeking relief from back pain.

As proof that both local and distal acupuncture points can be effective in treating back pain, these are the points of the body where acupuncture was used during this particular study:

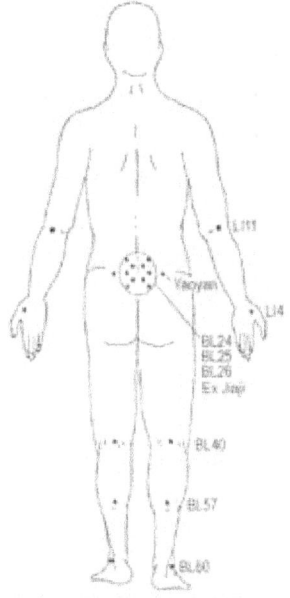

Figure II: Acupuncture points used in the study. Points are labeled according to World Health Organization standards.

Chiropractic Manipulation

In some cases, visiting a chiropractor for manipulation of the area of the body where pain is being felt can be effective.

Indeed, chiropractic manipulation can in certain circumstances be every bit as effective as medical (i. e. pharmaceutical drug based) treatment for a back pain condition.

It is however extremely important to understand that chiropractic manipulation is not going to be effective in every situation, and that in certain circumstances, it could even make your back pain problem considerably worse, depending upon the root cause of that problem.

Indeed, if your back pain problem is a result of spinal damage, for example, using a chiropractor to reduce your back pain could actually be extremely dangerous.

For this reason, you must have an x-ray to establish whether you have any spinal damage or instability before considering using a chiropractor as a way of reducing your back pain.

In addition, if you have pain in other areas that might be associated with a back problem (e. g. in your buttocks or legs) or any other neurologic condition (e. g. numbness or tingling), you should seek qualified medical advice before considering visiting a chiropractor for treatment.

Massage For Back Pain

Many people find that enjoying a good massage will help to alleviate their back pain problems, although it should be noted that this relief is often relatively temporary.

However, if massage is capable of providing back pain relief, then the only thing that you have to lose by visiting a masseur is the money that it is going to cost you to do so.

Furthermore, it is also necessary to take the same precautions as you would before visiting a chiropractor if you are considering visiting a masseur to seek relief from your back pain problems.

Herbs For Back Pain

Current research suggests that depression and stressful events can make pain worse, meaning that chronic pain sufferers are likely to respond to depression or stress with more pain. Consequently, this research suggests that substances which can calm and soothe your nervous system will therefore also help to relieve your pain.

For this reason, herbs that can reduce your stress levels are likely to be highly effective aids in your fight against back pain. Included in this category would be skullcap, valerian, St John's wort, poppy, willow bark, angelica, cayenne, wild yam, motherwort, rose and lavender.

In addition, the essential oils of peppermint, pine, rosemary, frankincense, ginger, cloves or juniper can be used as pain killers because every one of them has recognized analgesic qualities. Infuse one liquid ounce of a suitable carrier oil like olive or coconut oil with 10-12 drops of any of these essential oils, shake well and then rub the oil on the skin in the area of back pain. This will alleviate the pain and also reduce any swelling or inflammation.

If you have chronic back pain, try to drink a few cups of skullcap infusion every day, or alternatively take a dozen or so drops of skullcap tincture every day. Alternatively, a mixture of equal parts of the skullcap tincture, St John's wort and oat straw is known to be particularly effective for calming the nerves, and that will have a knock- on effect in helping to alleviate chronic back pain.

St John's wort oil can be liberally rubbed into any area of your back in which you feel pain, and as it is a particularly effective treatment for muscular pain, this can be an extremely valuable antidote to chronic or acute muscular back pain.

Yoga To Deal With Back Pain

Contrary to popular and mistaken belief, yoga is not simply a form of exercise or something that is only focused on striking certain poses. Instead, yoga is primarily focused on teaching devotees to adopt a total balanced approach to life, taking in both physical exercise and mental adaptability and adroitness.

Most importantly for any back pain sufferer, yoga lays great emphasis on body alignment, and it is often the fact that peoples bodies are forced into positions where it is not correctly aligned that causes back pain in the first place.

For example, if you spend many hours everyday sitting at your desk working on a computer, or behind the wheel of your car driving, you are putting your body into a position which is almost inevitably going to cause stress to develop in your back. Consequently, even though there is no one single event or situation that causes you to suffer back pain, the daily misalignment of your body is inevitably going to cause back problems eventually.

There are many reasons why yoga is likely to be far more effective as a form of exercise for alleviating or reducing your back when compared to other forms of exercise.

In the first place, because yoga places a great deal of emphasis on the spiritual side of practicing, the controlled breathing or pranayama techniques that you learn when studying yoga are an essential part of the practice. Deep, slow breathing naturally relaxes your muscles, which will obviously reduce the chances of suffering a muscle strain or sprain in the first place, and alleviate the pain if you have already caused a strain.

On top of this, yogic asanas or poses are all about stretching all the muscles in your body, and this also makes it far less likely that you will suffer strains or muscle damage in the future.

As a result, yoga has two functions as far as back pain is concerned. In the first place, it can reduce the pain that you may already be suffering by making you more flexible and supple, while it can also prevent back problems developing if you are not already a back pain sufferer.

The fact is, if you do not already take regular exercise, whether that is jogging, swimming, cycling or even walking, your spine will have become more rigid and less flexible. It is far more likely that you will suffer back damage the next time you make any significant demands on your back.

This is not to say that you should take up a rigorous or strenuous sporting activity immediately, because doing so is as likely to damage your back as it is to strengthen it.

Yoga is the perfect solution, because, while it is excellent for improving your flexibility and suppleness, it is not an exercise form that is as potentially harmful as many others might be. For example, while jogging might appear to be a relatively simple and benign form of exercise, the running action is relatively high impact as your feet pound the road or sidewalk, and this impact can very quickly 'announce' itself as lower back pain.

Nevertheless, if you are thinking of taking up yoga either to alleviate existing back pain or to prevent a future back pain problem, you should consult your regular medical attendant to confirm that it is okay to do so before starting. While it is not as immediately stressful or strenuous a form of exercise as many others, yoga is nevertheless exercise, and you need medical confirmation that you are up to the task before embarking on yogic training.

It would also be highly advisable that you start training under the professional supervision of a suitably qualified yoga teacher. While there are many websites that present pictorial illustrations of the asanas (poses) that are most widely recognized to be 'back-friendly', it will certainly be safer and probably more productive for you to learn these poses properly from the outset.

To be fair, some of the poses that are most commonly recommended for back pain sufferers would not appear to be that difficult to master, such as the 'Balasana' pose ('Child pose') taken from the *Yoga Cards* website:

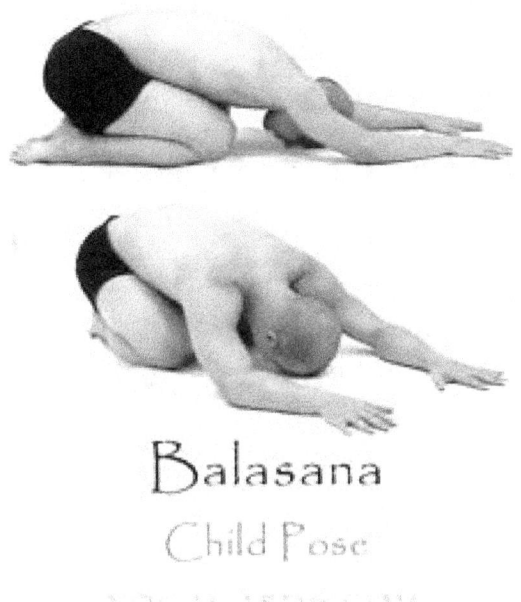

Balasana

Child Pose

Nevertheless, there are subtleties even in a seemingly simple pose such as this one which you are unlikely to discover on your own, and therefore seeking professional advice and training is definitely recommended.

In addition to the Yoga cards website, you might also want to look at some of the articles about yoga and back pain listed by *about. com*, study some of the recommended poses from the same site and read some of the back pain relief extracts from '*Yoga for Wellness*' here.

Back Mobility Exercises

Even if you are still in some pain there are back mobility exercises that will give you relief and when your back is normal again these back mobility exercises will ensure that your back muscles become (and remain) strong.

Initially if you are in pain it is recommended that you consider aquatic therapy to help with your back mobility. There are plenty of videos on the net that will demonstrate the techniques but the best one, we think, can be found at this web address https://www.youtube.com/watch?v=mVvzsFk6rPo

The best back mobility exercise videos we have come across are from Dr. Neil King, an eminent chiropractor. You can view his videos here

http://www.monkeysee.com/play/7302-low-back-and-hip-mobility-exercises

As always we urge you to consult your medical practitioner about the suitability of these exercises for you before performing the exercises.

Conclusion

As you have read in this book, there are many ways that you can deal with back pain without resorting to pharmaceutical chemicals or drugs.

In addition, there are many simple lifestyle changes that you can make that will significantly reduce the chances of you ever suffering back pain in the future, and you should consider adopting those changes which are most appropriate to your current lifestyle or situation.

Undoubtedly, the single most important thing that you should keep in mind now that you have finished reading is that treating your back pain in a natural manner should always be the number one choice, and that there is no need whatsoever for dealing with your back pain naturally to be difficult. After all, it is hard to imagine anything more natural or indeed simple than making sure that you sleep in a bed which does not make your back pain problem any worse.

From a personal point of view, I would thoroughly recommend that anyone who suffers from a back pain problem should take up yoga, because there is no doubt whatsoever that doing so will significantly help to deal with your back pain.

Apart from paying for a few yoga classes, it is also something that you can do at no cost in the privacy of your own home, and at any time you like. In addition, I would say that the extra strength and flexibility that you would naturally acquire by practicing yoga would almost certainly mean that your back pain problems would become a thing of the past.

The central point is, your back pain problems can be dealt with entirely naturally, and after reading this book, you now know how.

All that therefore remains is for you to start putting what you have just learned into practice so that back pain becomes something that only ever happens to other people (those that do not have this book, that is)!

www.ingramcontent.com/pod-product-compliance
Lightning Source LLC
Chambersburg PA
CBHW070842290526
45795CB00002B/952